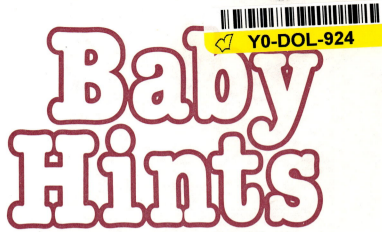

Baby Hints

By Chris Casson Madden
Illustrations by Greg Metcalf

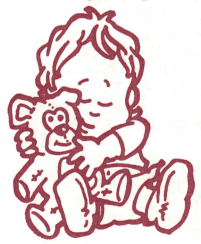

Mary Ellen Enterprises

BABY HINTS
Mary Ellen Enterprises
6414 Cambridge Street
St. Louis Park, MN 55426-4461
Copyright © 1982 by Mary Ellen Enterprises, Inc.
ALL RIGHTS RESERVED
ISBN: 0-941298-05-1
Printed in the United States of America
First Printing: April 1982
10   9   8   7   6   5   4   3   2   1

Created and Designed by Mary Ellen Enterprises
Art Director: **Tom Oberg**
Poetry: **Lydia Wilen**

This Book Is Dedicated To
Each and Every Miracle Maker!

Contents

INTRODUCTION BY
Mary Ellen

When I was pregnant, a friend gave me some hand-me-down baby clothes. I went through the bundle and, in order to fix up a few of the things, I took out some dental floss, an electric razor and a box of electric dishwasher detergent. My friend thought I was off my rocker. Then I sewed on some buttons with the dental floss. (The garments may fall apart, but the buttons will stay on forever!) I shaved off all the fuzzies from a sweet little sweater, using the electric razor. And, the electric dishwasher detergent was used to get those little white cotton T-shirts white again.

If my friend had read this book, she would have known all about those things and more: Running diaper pins through one's hair; suspenders for the crib sheet; marbles for cleaning baby bottles; and, how to recycle playpens.

This book can make life with your baby a little easier and lots more fun. It encourages your creativity and offers advice that would be new to your mother, your best friend, and your doctor.

Carl Sandburg said, "A baby is God's opinion that the world should go on." How nice to share that thought with you parents and parents-to-be. Bless you and your babies!   **Mary Ellen Pinkham**

i

Diaper Data

When it comes to diapering baby
It really isn't an art
Just read this chapter, then—
BOTTOMS UP!
That's the place to start

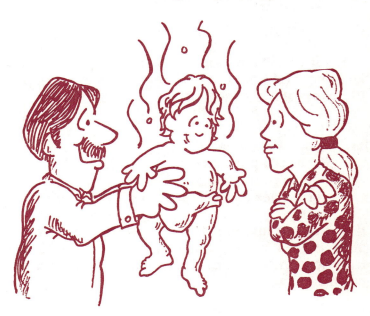

DIAPERS:
THE ETERNAL TRIANGLE

Nothing beats a disposable
- Disposable diapers are best when you get home from the hospital. You'll need your time to rest instead of washing diapers.

Disposables on the mend
- When the tab on a disposable diaper pulls off or will not stick, use masking tape.

- Or, in a pinch, use a band-aid.

- When it can't be repaired, remove the plastic backing and use the liner with another disposable. It's perfect for overnight or traveling.

Disposables do more
- Use one as a lap protector.

- Or, as shoulder protection at burping time.

- If you're nursing and find you need extra protection at times, remove the tapes and cut disposable diapers into sections. The protective lining will keep your clothing dry.

It's a boy!

- For better coverage on a boy, you may want to put the diaper on backwards. Now, the diaper will be higher on baby's stomach, absorbing more moisture and providing a better fit.

- When using a disposable diaper, fold the front of the diaper down inside to prevent wet tummy and clothes.

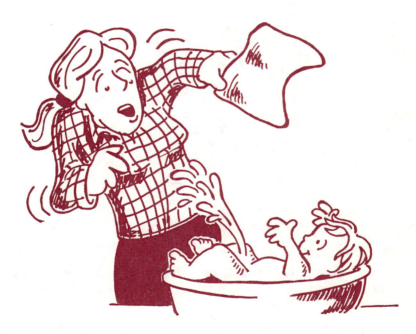

Fountain of youth

- To avoid being squirted, cover a boy with a cloth as you change him.

3

It's a girl!

- Lay a disposable diaper under your daughter when changing her. It will keep what's underneath dry.

- For special occasions, put fancy panties over a disposable under baby's dress and she'll be all dolled up.

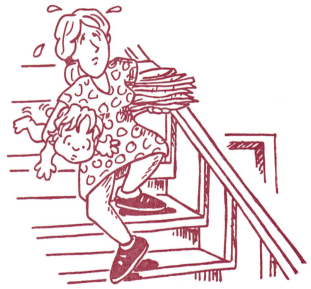

The changing place

- Save a lot of legwork if you live in a two-story house by keeping diaper-changing supplies on both floors.

- The bathroom vanity is a handy place to change diapers. Lay baby on a towel with her "tushy" near the edge of the sink. Now splash warm water on baby's bottom with water from the basin.

- Or, turn a sturdy card table into a changing table. Put a plastic foam pad on top and cover the sides with an attractive skirt. Use the area under the table for storage.

Do-it-yourself diapers
- Save money! Buy 10 yards of diaper flannel to make a dozen diapers. Cut a starter slash in the flannel and tear it across the grain to the length you want. The flannel will ravel a little, but will stop after a few washings.

- To prevent leaks, take a tuck at the back of each leg and fasten with a piece of masking tape.

Handy additions
- A bicycle basket fastened to the end of the crib makes a handy place to keep diapers, lotions and pins. When baby gets older, remove the basket.

- A towel rack installed on the outside of a crib makes a good place to hang extra blankets and clothing.

- Or, hang clothes on a wooden accordion-like mug rack near the changing area.

A happy baby is easy to change
- A securely hung mirror beside baby's changing table gives your baby a "friend" to talk to while you make the change.

- Or, paste pictures of happy babies on the wall next to the changing table.

Baby powder

- Instead of shaking on baby powder, pour a little in the palm of your hand and smooth it over your baby's skin. Baby powder can be harmful to the lungs, and this helps prevent either of you from breathing too much of it.

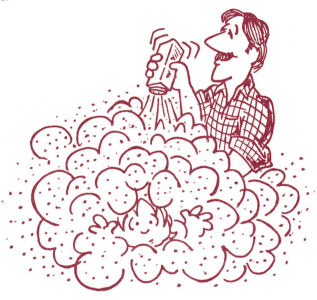

- Or, put powder in a large bath powder box and apply with a powder puff.

- Use cornstarch as an inexpensive substitute for baby powder.

- Or, if you like the scent of baby powder, mix in an equal amount of cornstarch.

6

Dull diaper pins
- Run them through your hair. The oils will lubricate the pins and they will go through the material easily.

- Or, stick them into a wrapped bar of soap. Just make sure the soap is out of baby's reach.

Remember
- Never hold diaper pins in your mouth. Baby might imitate Mommy.

Traveling pins
- Attach a few diaper pins to your key chain. You'll always have extras when you're away from home.

Handy wiping
- Place folded paper towels or napkins into a small container. Pour in some water and add a couple splashes of baby oil. You've just made your own baby wipes. (Keep the container tightly closed.)

- Or, use worn-out diapers that have been cut into squares. Baby wipes that can be laundered!

- If you keep a washcloth and a pump Thermos bottle filled with warm water near your changing table, there will be no need to run to the sink.

Oil change
- Your hands won't get greasy when applying baby oil if you transfer the oil into clean, empty roll-on antiperspirant bottle. (To remove the roller ball, pry it off gently with a nail file.)

Rash moves

- To help prevent and treat diaper rash, change diapers as soon as possible—even throughout the night.

- If you've been using cloth diapers, switch to disposables or see "Eight ounces of prevention" (below).

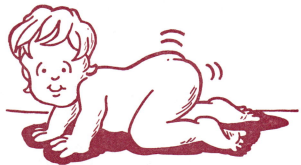

- Let baby stay bare-bottomed as often as possible. This is a nuisance, but exposure to air is the best treatment.

- Drying with a cloth may cause further irritation to baby's sensitive skin. Instead, dry baby's bottom with warm (not hot) air from a non-asbestos hair dryer after each change. Be sure to hold it at least six inches from the skin.

- To avoid chafing already-reddened skin, splash baby's bottom with warm water instead of wiping with a cloth.

Eight ounces of prevention

- Add 1 cup of white distilled vinegar to the final rinse cycle when washing diapers. This will remove all detergent and ammonia which can cause diaper rash.

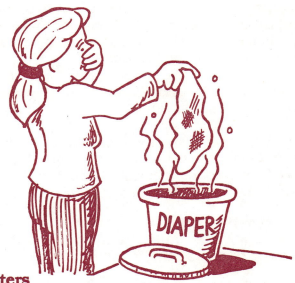

Odor eaters
- Deodorize the diaper pail by placing a few charcoal briquets under the plastic trash bag used to hold disposable diapers. Change briquets every week.

- Or, sprinkle baking soda into the pail.

- Deodorizers that stick to the diaper pail lid sometimes fall inside and get thrown away accidentally. To prevent this, put the deodorizer inside an old nylon knee-high sock, tie the open end to the pail handle, and hang the deodorizer inside.

Wash day the right way
- After soaking diapers in a diaper pail, spin out the excess water in the washing machine before laundering.

- For extra-clean diapers, soak them overnight in the washing machine. Pour in 1 cup of Ivory Snow and 1 cup bleach or a commercial soaking preparation. In the morning, run the diapers through the entire cycle.

- It's a good idea to run diapers through an extra rinse cycle. Soap residue can cause skin irritation.

- Keep diapers soft and fresh-smelling by adding a half-cup of baking soda at the beginning of the washing cycle. Fabric softener can irritate tender skin. Besides, too much softness reduces absorbency.

Care of plastic pants
- If plastic pants become dry and crinkly, add some baby oil to the rinse water.

- Do not put plastic pants in your dryer. If you need them right away, dry with a hair blow-dryer.

- Or, hang them on a multiple skirt hanger out in the sun. Sunlight kills odors.

- Add baking soda to the wash water to help rid them of odors.

Inside clothesline
- When drying diapers indoors, space may be a problem. But not if you hang two coat hangers on your shower curtain rod so they are parallel. Pin one corner of a diaper to one hanger, and the other corner to the other hanger. Fill up the hangers and it's just like two short clotheslines, side by side.

Open Up Wide

Here comes the plane so open wide
I'm going to put something yummy inside.
Broccoli and squash with vitamins galore
Whoops!
We're going to have the healthiest floor!

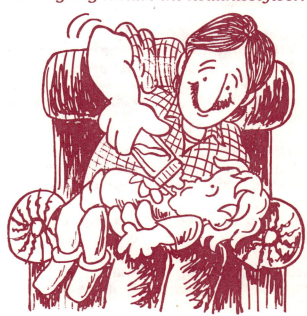

BOTTLE FEEDING

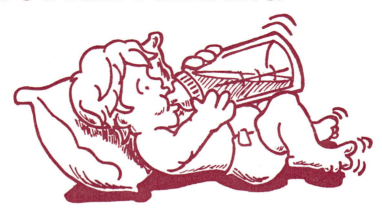

The formula for using formula
- Check the expiration date on the can before you buy it, and check it again before you use it.

- Before opening the can, wash the top and rinse it thoroughly.

- Follow the instructions precisely as printed on the can. Diluting too much or too little throws off the carefully determined nutritional balance of the formula.

- Stir powder preparations enough to eliminate all lumps.

Preparing and storing formula
- Be sure to refrigerate the formula after you've sterilized it.

- Once you've opened canned formula, cover it with aluminum foil or plastic wrap before storing in the refrigerator.

- Or, cover the opened can with a clean plastic lid from a can of chocolate syrup.

- NEVER freeze formula. It will separate.

Regulating the flow
- If the formula flows too slowly, loosen the rim of the bottle slightly. Tighten it if it flows too quickly.

- Hold the bottle at feeding angle to check if the hole in the nipple is the right size. If the formula comes out in steady, even drops, the nipple is ready to use.

- If the nipple hole has to be enlarged, stick a very hot needle into it a few times until the rubber widens.

Early morning feedings
- If it's a hassle to get up and go all the way to the kitchen, put the bottle in an insulated ice bucket in your baby's room before going to bed. And fill the bottom of an electric coffee pot with a few inches of water to use as a bottle warmer.

- For a fast warmup, put a cold, uncapped bottle without the nipple in the microwave for 30 to 60 seconds.

- Or, leave a Thermos bottle filled with boiling water in the kitchen before going to bed.

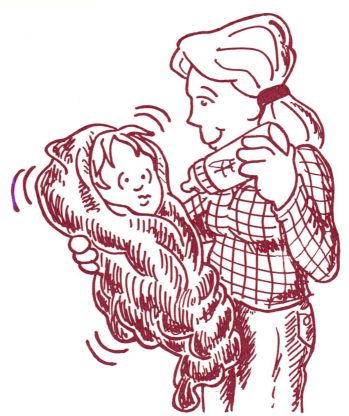

All wrapped up
- If baby is extremely active and just about wriggles out of your arms during feedings, wrap a terrycloth towel snuggly around her. She'll be much easier to hold.

Too hot?
- Keep extra formula on hand in the refrigerator to add to a bottle of formula that's too hot.

Just right!

- Formula will heat up evenly if you give the bottle a few good shakes while it's warming on the stove. Use a pot holder to protect your hands.

Nipple know-how

- Before sterilizing, make sure nipples aren't clogged. Simply fill them with water and squeeze it through the nipple hole with your finger.

- When nipples are clogged and gummy, put them in a pan of water, add a teaspoon of baking soda and boil for several minutes. After they have been rinsed and dried, store them in a glass jar with a lid.

- To sterilize nipples in the microwave, add a teaspoon of vinegar to a glass jar filled with water.

- Wash nipples in the dishwasher by hanging them from the top rack inside a nylon mesh bag. This way, they won't scatter or damage the machine.

- A clean berry basket is just the right size to drain and dry bottle caps, nipples and seals.

Bottle business

- Cleanse plastic bottles of sour milk smell by filling with warm water and adding 1 teaspoon of baking soda to each. Shake well and let set overnight before washing in soap and hot water.

- When cleaning bottles, place a few agate marbles in the sterilizer or sauce pan to gather the corrosion.

- Sterilize bottles by washing them on the lower rack of your dishwasher.

Formula residue
- That chalky residue that forms in bottles can be removed by boiling for 10 minutes in a pan of water to which 1 cup of vinegar has been added.

Introducing juice
- Serve juices at room temperature. They lose some vitamin value if heated, and cold juice can be a shock to a baby's system.

- If baby isn't crazy about juice, dilute it with water while he's getting used to the new taste.

Fruit-juice stains
- Fill the stained bottle with hot water and add a teaspoon of automatic dishwasher detergent. Shake well and let stand; then give the bottle a few more shakes every 15 minutes or so until the stain has loosened. Rinse thoroughly in hot water.

More bottle business
- Save a couple of empty soft drink cartons and use them to hold baby bottles in the refrigerator. The bottles will be easier to move and won't get knocked over.

- Having your friends and their babies over for a visit? To avoid mix-ups, mark your bottles with strips of tape.

- You'll be able to tell at a glance how much formula has been taken if you paint the ounce marks on the outside of plastic bottles with red nail polish.

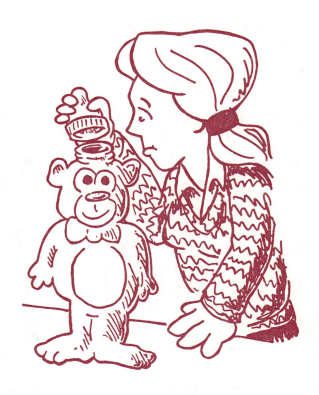

- Steer clear of fun-shaped plastic bottles. They're no fun at all when it comes to keeping them clean.

Burping

- The standard method works almost everytime. Put a diaper on your shoulder and the baby on top of it. Gently pat her back between her shoulder blades.

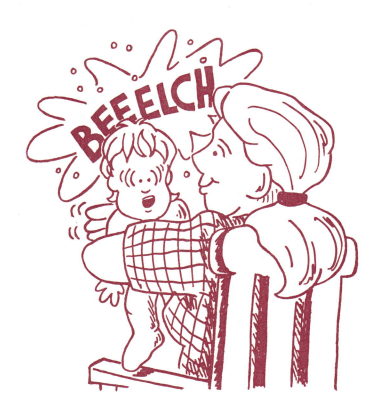

- Or, cover your lap with a diaper or towel and place the baby on it, face down. Gently massage her back, or pat it.

- Or, sit with the baby on your lap, facing you. Tilt her backward slightly while your hand supports her head and back. This position alone may help release the bubble. If not, pat gently.

Going off the bottle

- When the time has come to drink from a cup, but baby refuses, try taking the cap and nipple off the bottle and let him drink from that until you can ease him into a cup.

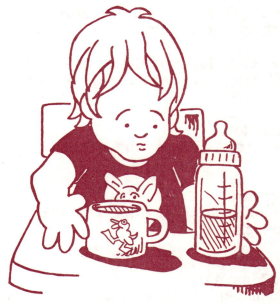

- .Or, put his favorite drinks in a cup and his least favorite drinks in the bottle, Soon, he'll want everything in the cup.

Getting a grip on glasses

- A few strips of adhesive tape around a drinking glass provide a steadier grip for tiny hands.

- Or, cover the bottom of the glass with the ribbing of an old sock.

BREAST FEEDING

Where do I start?

- Use a large diaper pin on your nursing bra to remind you which side to start.

- Or, switch a ring from the finger of one hand to the finger of the other hand to help you keep track.

Extra comfort

- Use a bedrest when feeding in bed.

Mommy care

- Make sure to drink juice, water or milk right after nursing to replace liquid.

Storing Mom's milk

- Extra milk can be stored in boilable pouches. Seal it, date it and freeze it. When needed, drop a pouch of frozen milk into a pan of hot water. (Mother's milk should last three to four months in the freezer.)

All that glitters

- Remove dangle or hoop earrings when nursing or feeding. They won't be temptations for little hands.

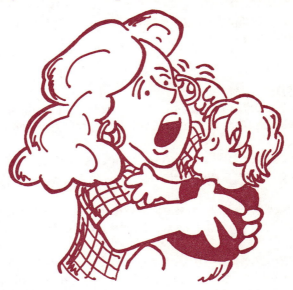

- If you have long hair, put it in a ponytail.

INTRODUCING SOLID FOOD

In the beginning

- The first solid food will probably be rice cereal mixed into the formula. If you give it to him in a bottle, first run it through the blender and the cereal will pass through the nipple hole easier.

- Introduce a new food at the start of the meal, when he's hungriest.

- Start him on only one new food a week. That way, if there are any allergic reactions, you can pinpoint the cause easily.

His Nib's bib
- Tuck a few sponges in the pocket of a plastic bib. The pocket stays open and absorbs the spilled liquid.

- For better bib coverage, safety-pin the bottom of the bib to baby's clothes.

- He won't get as messy if you tuck a double thickness of tissue under the neckline to catch the drools.

- Make one big bib by snapping two terry cloth bibs together front-to-back. When one side becomes messy, just rotate the bib.

- Protect long-sleeved shirts from food stains by covering the arms with the ribbing from an old pair of gym socks.

Baby's dish-position
- When baby thinks he's big enough to eat from a plate, give him a plastic plate with a raised rim to hold spills to a minimum.

- Or, if baby has a habit of knocking his dish on the floor, buy a plastic dish with a rubber suction cup on the bottom.

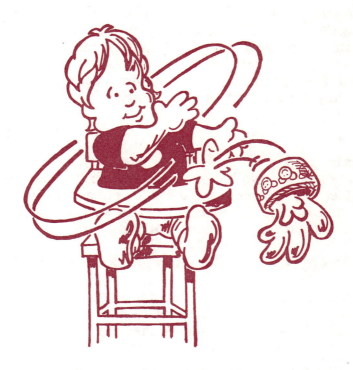

- Or, buy plastic cups with weighted bottoms.

Another sticky problem
- Remove sticky food from baby's face by rubbing the area gently with petroleum jelly.

Spoon feeding
- Demitasse spoons are perfect for baby. Or, use a sugar spoon.

- As he grows older, give him his own spoon to play with while you feed him with another spoon. Soon, he'll start copying you and learn to feed himself.

- Remember, mashed potatoes are a good training food. They don't fall off a spoon easily.

Fixin' food
- Make your own baby food. Puree fresh-cooked vegetables in your blender, place in ice-cube trays and freeze; then transfer to airtight freezer bags. Make sure you mark the bag as to contents and date.

- An egg poacher is ideal to warm foods all at once.

- Or, put the meal in a divided frying pan.

- Add a little liquid to soft-cooked meats so they'll grind easier in the baby food grinder.

This'll fool 'em!
- If your youngster balks at vegetables or fruit, puree them and add to gelatin. It's a good way to slip in some nutrition.

Loosening a tight lid

- If the screw-top on a baby food jar won't budge, punch a hole (carefully!) in the top with an ice pick. This releases the vacuum inside the jar and the lid will unscrew easily.

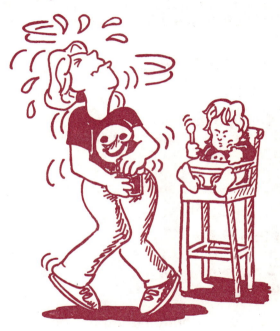

- Never spoon feed straight from the jar, you'll be introducing bacteria to the unused portion. Remove the amount you think he will eat and refrigerate the rest.

- A two-tiered lazy Susan is perfect for storing all those baby food jars in your pantry. It holds a week's supply of food, and one spin tells you what's in stock.

High on highchairs

- A highchair won't tip over if you attach it to the wall with a screen door hook and eye latch.

- To the back or side of the highchair, attach a small-sized towel rack to hold all things needed at mealtime such as a bib, washcloth and towel.

- Clean chrome and plastic highchairs in a hot shower or outside with a garden hose.

Under the highchair

- Lay a large trash bag under the highchair to catch spills.

- Or, use a washable shower curtain.

Slip-sliding away

- Pad the back of the highchair with bath towels to prevent baby from slipping down. This also provides added support while he sits.

- A thick foam rubber cushion on the seat of the highchair will prevent baby from sliding down. It also keeps spilled liquids from running onto the floor.

- A small rubber sink mat on the seat of the highchair also works.

All Quiet on the Nursery Front

Everything is worthwhile trying
Just to stop baby's crying
A bottle, a burp, or a pacifier
What will hush my little crier?
Sing lullabies, read fairy tales
To control the Prince of Wails
The real solution for all those tears?
Oh, about nine, ten or eleven years!

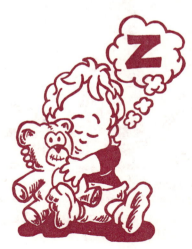

SLEEP LIKE A BABY

Mommy's scent

- Dab on your favorite perfume before the nurse brings the baby in for feedings. Not only will it make you feel good, but your newborn will get to know the "Mommy scent". Then, once you're home, dab a little perfume on the crib sheet. The familiar scent will be a comfort at night.

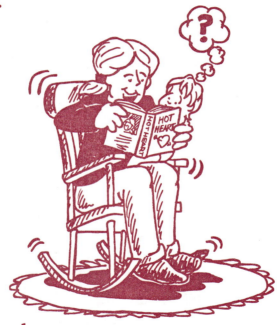

Sandman schemes

- While rocking the baby, read your favorite novel aloud to her. She'll think you're talking to her while you catch up on your reading.

28

- Be aware of sounds that are soothing, such as running water (which simulates intrauterine sounds) or the hum of an air conditioner. Tape the sound, play it at bedtime and let it lull her to sleep.

A little night music
- A radio turned on low might help her make it through the night. After a few weeks, decrease the volume. Then, turn it off completely when the baby is feeling more secure.

- Or, try whistling a tune directly in her face. The soft stream of air will encourage her to shut her eyes, while the melody lulls her to sleep.

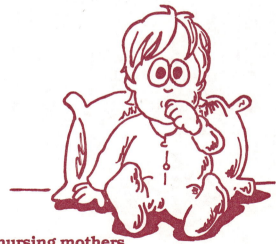

Note to nursing mothers
- If your baby has trouble sleeping, watch what you eat! Limit caffeine products such as coffee, tea, cola drinks, and chocolate.

Bedside manner
- Stick to the same nightly going-to-sleep rituals like closing the curtains, winding up a musical toy, patting baby's back while singing a song, or reciting a poem.

Warm thoughts
- Keep a heating pad or hot water bottle handy so you can warm the crib. Wouldn't you settle down faster on a nice, toasty bed? Make sure you remove the heating pad and test the bedding before putting baby on it.

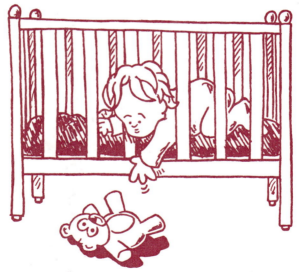

Bumper pads
- They keep off drafts, prevent toys from slipping through the slats and are often a comfort to babies who can't sleep unless their heads are up against something.

30

Crib sheets

- For quick, middle-of-the-night changes, make up the crib using two or more crib sheets with rubberized flannel pads in between. You need only remove the top sheet and pad and the crib is ready again.

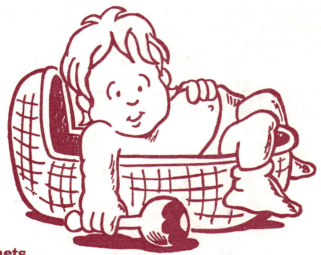

Bassinets

- Baby outgrows a bassinet in a few months. Instead of going through the expense of a new, store-bought one, be creative. Redecorate an old wicker basket with a coat of non-toxic paint, some ribbons, a few fabric flowers and a little imagination. Cut foam rubber to fit the basket's base and you have a one-of-a-kind bassinet.

- Don't go to the expense of buying a bassinet if you've already got a baby carriage. Or, if you have the choice between the two, buy the carriage. It will double as a traveling bassinet.

Bassinet sheets
- Use pillowcases as sheets for the bassinet.

Some light on the subject
- An adorable novelty lamp in the nursery is fine, but an overhead light controlled by a dimmer switch is much more convenient and flexible. You can check on the baby in a very dim light without waking him; when you need a bright light, you'll have that, too.

- Or, keep a flashlight next to your bed for middle-of-the-night bedchecks.

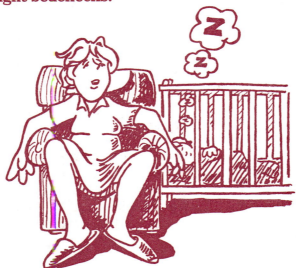

Nursery extras
- If there's room, put a big, comfortable chair in the nursery. You may spend a lot of time there the first few months.

- A folding cot is a welcome addition, especially if you're nursing, or for when baby is sick.

Night moves
- If your baby insists on night feedings, play it down. Don't turn on the lights or make any unnecessary motions to make him think it's time to get up.

Rise and shine — but not too early
- After your toddler falls asleep, put a couple of toys in her crib. When she awakens and finds them, she may be distracted long enough to let you get some early-morning sleep.

- If your toddler begins to wake up too early, put a clock radio in her room and tell her to play until the radio comes on. Gradually increase playtime (and your sleep time) from 15 minutes the first week, to a half-hour the second week, and so on.

Nap happy
- When a newborn naps, you should try to nap, too. Why? It may be quite a while before you get a night of eight uninterrupted hours sleep!

Daytime naps
- Put baby in a carriage or playpen for daytime naps. That will reinforce the message that the crib is for a full night's sleep.

No interruptions
- A picture of a sleeping baby hung by the nursery door will let others know that the baby is sleeping.

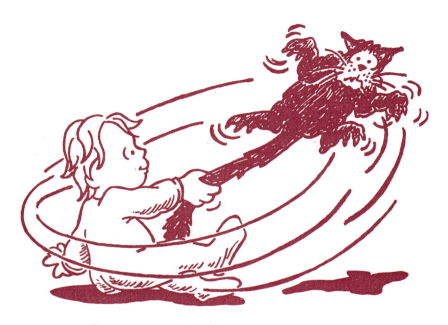

Pet-proof nursery
- Install a screen door. It will keep out the dog or cat, and you'll be able to check on baby without disturbing her.

Let Ma Bell tell
- A telephone answering machine can act as a secretary when you and baby are napping. Your message can be the birth announcement.

- Or, if you don't want to be disturbed during the nap time, put the phone on a soft pillow. You'll hear it ring if you're awake, but it won't disturb your sleep.

Sound advice
- When baby's asleep, don't talk in whispers or tip-toe around for fear of waking him. Let him hear the natural noises of his home. He'll begin to feel more secure with the sounds and he won't be conditioned to wake every time a pin drops.

THE BAWL GAME

For crying out loud
- Some babies simply need to cry themselves to sleep. There's nothing wrong with it and there's no reason for you to feel guilty.

Tapering off the tears
- Motion helps sometimes. Take baby for a short ride in a stroller or carriage.

- Or, try the mirror trick. A baby looking at his own image may be distracted long enough to stop crying.

- Put a warm hot-water bottle on your lap. Lay him across it and gently massage his arms and legs.

- A noisy toy, like a rattle, will work sometimes.

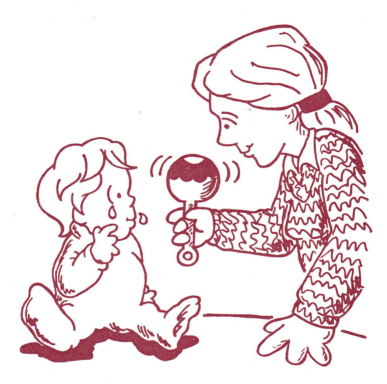

- Give him a loving hug while breathing slowly and calmly. If you're calm, he may become calm.

It's only a bad dream
- If your toddler seems to be having a nightmare and he won't stop crying, wash his face with lukewarm water. This will waken him fully and he can more easily be comforted.

This is a recording

- Some babies may be calmed by playing back a tape recording of their own sounds and cries. Even at a very young age, they are apparently able to distinguish the sound of their own voice and be quieted by it. Be careful with this hint, though. You don't want to stop crying that is caused by hunger or wet diapers.

Down falls

- When your child is learning to walk, don't make a big fuss if she falls down occasionally and starts to cry. If you give her too much attention, she'll cry at every spill.

Last resort

- Call a friend or relative who is willing to sit for a few hours while you get out of the house. Simply getting away from the crying may help you cope with it better.

ON YOUR BEST BEHAVIOR

Thumb sucking

- It's possible that baby requires extra sucking time during feedings and, for that reason, sucks her thumb. If that's the case, make feedings last a minimum of 15 to 20 minutes. You may have to change the type of nipple to slow down the rate of flow.

Breaking the pacifier habit

- Each week, cut off a little piece of the pacifier until it's gone.

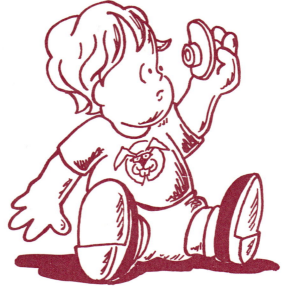

- Try dunking the pacifier in sauerkraut juice. That should do it.

- Or, tell your child that when the pacifier is worn out, that's it!

No! No! A thousand times, no!

- When the first and only word your child says is, "No!", you might be saying it too much. Listen to your own voice. Instead of telling your child what not to do, be positive and tell him what's better to do. You'll be surprised at the results!

Setting a good example

- Never encourage behavior that will have to be corrected in the future. For example, don't play with your child by letting her jump on the bed if this is something you don't want her to do later.

- On the other hand, when you want baby to get into a habit like spending time on the automatic swing or in the playpen, start as early as possible.

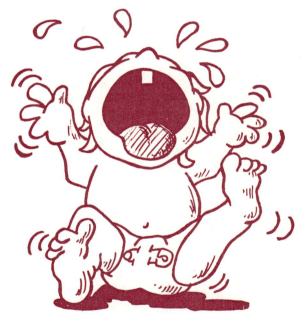

Temper tantrums

- When your toddler is screaming and seems uncontrollable, try whispering something in her ear. She may stop long enough to hear what you're whispering.

Laying down the law

- Bend down to eye level, look directly in your young-ster's eyes and speak in a low, controlled—but firm— voice. Make your statement in as few words as possible. "Don't kick!"; "Stay out of the driveway!"; "No jumping in puddles!"

- When you child does something wrong, make it clear that you disapprove of his behavior, but still approve of him.

Rub-A-Dub-Dub

Babies 'n' baths
Babies 'n' baths
How they kick and shout
First because they don't want in
Then they don't want out!

BABY'S IN THE TUB

To bathe or not to bathe

- Daily baths aren't necessary as long as you keep baby's bottom nice and clean. Three times a week is plenty.

- And, you don't have to shampoo more than twice a week.

- Give baths before feeding. Baby gets tired after eating.

Where to bathe?

- A kitchen sink or a bathroom vanity make great places to bathe. Choose an area that's warm and draft-free, with enough space for your bathing equipment.

Handy bath aids

- Bathtime won't be a slippery affair if you wear a pair of cotton gloves.

- Or, turn an old towel into a bath mitt. Trace your hand on an old towel, then cut and sew to form a mitt. Now you'll have a better grip on baby.

- Fill an empty dishwashing liquid bottle with baby shampoo and dilute with water. The pull-up top is less messy and more economical to use than a wide-mouth shampoo bottle.

- An inexpensive plastic apron is just the thing to hold shampoo, lotion, small tub toys and other bath needs.

- Wrap a bath towel around your neck and pin it on like a bib. It'll keep you dry and double as an after-bath wrap for baby.

In the tub
- Use an infant seat for bathing in the tub. After removing the pad, place a large towel on the seat and a rubber mat on the bathtub floor to prevent slipping. Now you can use both hands.

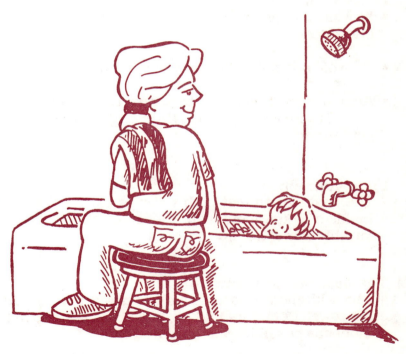

- Do your back a favor! Sit on a footstool next to the tub.

- Appliqués or decals glued to the tub floor will make it slip-proof.

- Or, us a rubber sink mat.

Go easy on the soap
- Soap depletes natural skin oils.

In the sink
- Prevent bumps on the head by turning the faucet to one side.

- To avoid slips, line the sink with a towel.

- After filling the sink or tub, turn the cold water off last. If there are any drips, little fingers or toes won't get burned.

Up to your elbow
- The best way to test bath water is to give it the old inside-of-your-elbow test. The water should be comfortably warm, not hot.

The best way to shampoo
- Line a kitchen counter or bathroom vanity with a Turkish towel. Put your child on it, face up, as close to the faucet as possible. Shampoo and rinse.

- Put a large sponge under her neck for comfort.

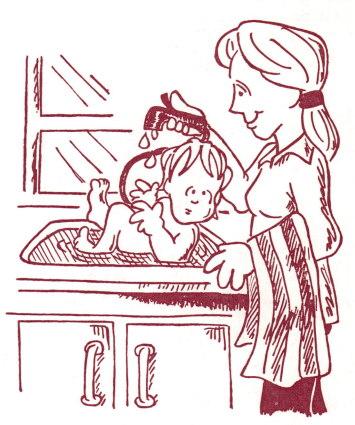

- For extra ease, attach a spray hose to the faucet.

'Tween sink and tub
- When baby is too big for the sink but afraid of the tub, compromise by using a plastic clothes basket with holes. Place the basket in the tub, run a few inches of water and set the baby inside the basket.

Comfort cloth

- If baby fusses in the bath, lay a washcloth over his tummy and pour warm water on it occasionally. He will relax in the warmth.

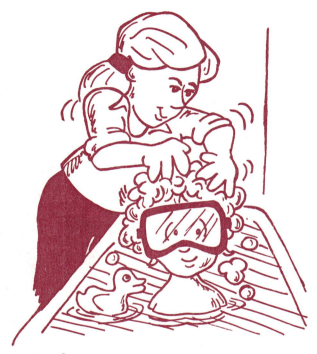

Fun ways to shampoo

- How about wearing a diving mask? It's fun and it will protect her eyes.

- Or, spread a little petroleum jelly over her eyebrows. This makes the soap run down her cheeks—not in her eyes.

- Have a mirror handy. She can watch as you shampoo her hair into funny styles.

Manicure-all
- Fingernails and toenails are soft and easy to clip right after the bath.

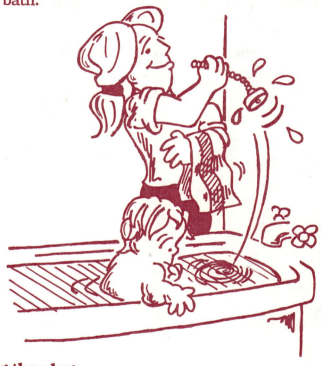

Pulling the plug
- If baby doesn't want to get out of the tub, pull the drain plug. Seeing the water disappear, he'll want to make a "clean" getaway.

After-bath aftermath

- Make the after-bath towel extra comfy by heating it on a radiator.

- Pat dry, don't rub tender skin.

- Warm a plastic container of lotion in the bath water during the bath.

- Be sparing with baby oil. Too much can clog pores.

Duds 'N' Suds

That pile of laundry
Is from my tiny little son
You'd think I'd had a litter
Instead of only one
I do two loads daily
To keep his clothes clean
God bless the inventor
Of the washing machine

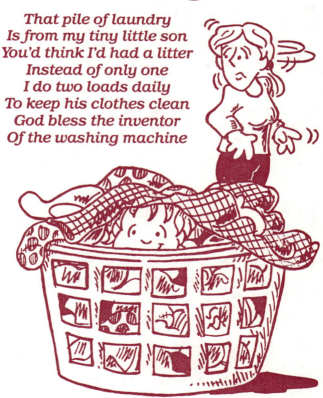

CLOTHES ENCOUNTERS

Make it easy on yourself
- Pants and overalls that have snap bottoms are more convenient when changing diapers.

When baby starts to crawl
- Put extra padding in the knees of baby's playsuit by patching them with pot holders. They help protect his knees as well as his clothing.

Saving and storing baby clothes
- To preserve a christening gown and other treasured baby clothes, store them in zip-lock bags. Squeeze as much air out as possible to keep the bag airtight and bug-proof.

- Keep a big box in baby's closet to store outgrown clothes.

- Save your little girl's baby clothes and use them to fill out her doll's wardrobe. Small and medium sizes will fit large dolls.

Longer lasting pj's
- Buy pajamas a size larger than needed and thread elastic through the hems at the wrists and ankles. As baby grows, remove the thread.

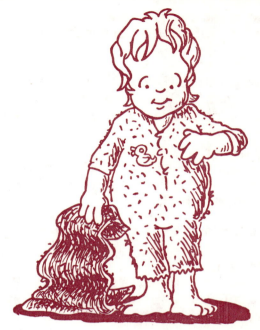

- Get more miles out of baby's favorite footy pajamas by snipping off the worn-out feet.

There's no escape
- Try dressing a wiggly toddler in the highchair. You'll have both arms free for socks, shoes and shirts.

The best buy
- Shop for little girl's play clothes in the boy's departments and save! Boy's clothes usually cost less and are made better.

Making the most out of dresses

- If a dress is too short, sew an edge of wide rickrack on the hem.

- Or, have your little girl wear the too-short dress over a coordinated pair of slacks as a smock top. Styles with high waistbands and raglan sleeves are perfect.

A growing jacket

- When the sleeves of a child's jacket become too short, lengthen them by sewing on knitted cuffs (available in notions departments).

- Or, cut off the jacket sleeves and make a vest.

Mitten minders

- To avoid lost mittens, sew a strip of VELCRO Fastener on mitten cuffs and corresponding strips on the inside of your child's coat cuffs.

- Or, sew a button to each mitten cuff and teach him to fasten them into button holes on his coat when he takes off his clothes.

- Or, crochet a woolen chain long enough to go through the toddler's coat sleeves and over his shoulders. Attach the mittens to the chain.

Nothing up my sleeve

- To prevent sweater sleeves from riding up when putting on a coat, sew an elastic loop inside your toddler's sweater cuff. Slip the loops over her thumbs, then slip on the coat.

Easy zipping

- Clip a notebook ring to a snowsuit zipper and it will be easier to pull.

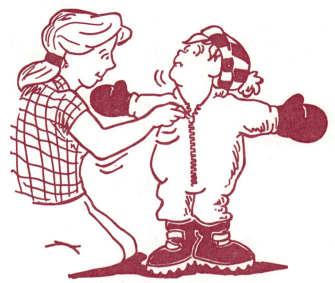

- Stuck zipper? Rub the zipper teeth with a lead pencil or a bar of soap.

Repairing drawstrings

- If toddler has pulled his drawstring out, wet it and place it in the freezer for a few minutes. When it's stiff it will be easy to insert in the hem.

- If you're tired of fishing for drawstrings in hoods or jackets, secure them into the hems with a few quick stitches.

A quick hem
- For instant repairs of toddler's dress slacks, tape up the hem with masking tape.

On the button
- Use dental floss or elastic thread to sew buttons on clothing. The buttons will take a lot of wear before falling off.

- Make those four-hole buttons last longer. Sew through two holes at a time, breaking the thread and knotting it for each pair. Should one set break, the other set will hold the button.

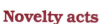

Novelty acts
- To keep iron-on novelty prints from fading or cracking on children's T-shirts and pajamas, soak in cold salt water before wearing.

- To repair a rip or tear in an iron-on decal, apply a few drops of nail polish with a toothpick, then gently close the edges of the rip. When the polish dries, the tear disappears.

Hanging around
- Use a tiered skirt hanger with clip hooks to hold shirts and pants. It saves time fumbling with small plastic hangers.

- Use an accordian-like mug rack as a coat rack in your youngster's room. Hang it low enough for him to reach. Soon he'll learn to hang up his own clothes.

In the closet
- Double the amount of closet space by adding a second clothing rod at tot height.

No closet?
- Suspend a hoola hoop toy from a plant hook with lengths of macrame so the hoop forms a flat, circular clothes rack.

SHOE BIZ

Lasting shines
- Spray shoes with hairspray after polishing to seal the shine.
- Or, shine with a transparent boot wax; then buff.

Patent leather

- Restore the shine to patent leather shoes by rubbing with petroleum jelly and a soft cloth.

- A black felt-tipped pen can be used to fill in little scrapes on patent leather shoes.

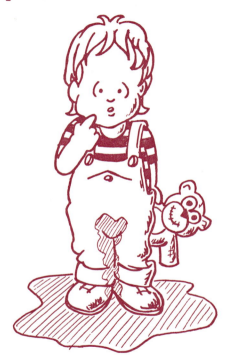

Wet shoes

- Puddle-soaked shoes won't become stiff if you rub them with saddle soap before they have dried. Allow to dry away from direct heat; then give them a good polishing.

- So that wet shoes don't lose their shape, stuff the toes with crumpled newspaper.

Sandy shoes
- Remove sand from the toes of baby shoes by brushing with a dry bottle brush.

Coping with canvas
- Spray children's sneakers with starch to keep them looking new.

- Clean sneakers with a scouring pad and soap. Rinse with lemon juice or bleach mixed with water.

- To quick-dry kid's tennis shoes, towel them off, then set your hair blow-dryer on high and place it inside each shoe for about five minutes. They should be dry enough to wear.

On a shoestring
- Tie knots at the ends of the laces after lacing your toddler's shoes. The shoes can be taken off, but the laces stay put.

- If laces are dampened before tying them, they'll stay tied.

- When the plastic tips wear off, replace them by coating the ends with clear nail polish.

- Or, wrap cellophane tape around the ends.

Tongue tied
- To prevent the tongues of your youngster's shoes from sliding down to one side, cut two parallel slits in each tongue. Pull the laces through the slots as you lace the shoes.

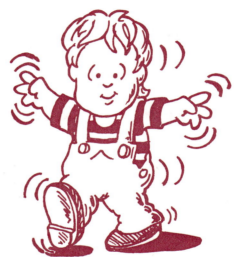

First steps
- With baby's first pair of hard-soled shoes, walking on a smooth surface is like walking on ice. Make the shoes less slippery by scraping the soles on sandpaper.

Ideas "to boot"
- Keep boots together when not in use with a clip-type clothespin.

- Inner-tube repair kits (available at hardware stores) are great for mending slashes or holes in rubber boots.

- Spray the inside of your children's boots with a furniture polish, then wipe the inside dry with a cloth. The boots will slip on and off much easier.

- Or, better yet, buy pull-on or snap-top boots so you won't have to struggle with zippers.

WASHING THE "LITTLE THINGS"

Dirty business
- To prevent dirt from grinding into the knees of a toddler's play clothes, spray starch on them.

- Help your child's dress clothes stay clean by spraying collars and cuffs with fabric protector.

Bag it
- Sew a simple nylon net drawstring bag and keep it near your changing table for little things that need to be washed. Put the clothes in the bag and toss it in the washer.

- Put baby's ribbon-trimmed dress in a mesh bag along with other delicate garments and wash in warm water, using light detergent and gentle action.

Baby's socks
- Dingy white socks will come clean again if they are soaked in a solution of washing soda before laundering.

Hat tricks
- Before a toddler wears a new knit cap and mittens, outline their shapes on cardboard and cut out the patterns. After washing the cap and mittens, slip the patterns inside the matching pieces. They'll dry in perfect shape.

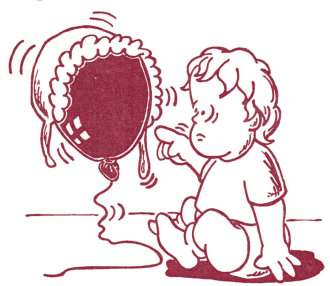

- A baby bonnet will keep its shape after washing if you let it dry on a blown-up balloon.

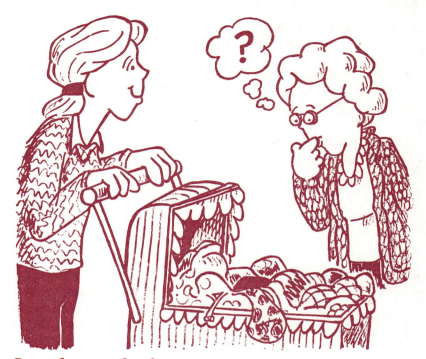

Laundry on wheels
- What to do with that outgrown bassinet or baby carriage? Line it with plastic and use it as a laundry basket on wheels.

Stain relievers
- Urine stains: Soak the stained garment for half an hour in a solution of 1 quart warm water, ½ teaspoon liquid dishwashing detergent and 1 tablespoon ammonia. Rinse, then put it through a wash.

- Baby food stains: Let the material soak for a few hours in a solution of 1 cup bleach, 1 cup dishwasher detergent and 2 to 3 gallons of water. Then wash.

- Formula stains: Try rubbing a paste of unseasoned meat tenderizer on formula stains. Roll the clothes up and wait a few hours before washing.

- Spit-up stains: To remove odor, apply a paste of baking soda in water to the fabric.

Better Safe Than Sorry

When baby starts to crawl on the floor
Make things safe for him to explore
There are precautions you shouldn't ignore
Read the following pages to find out more

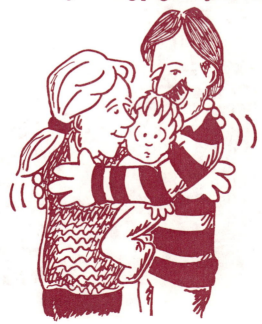

Babe's eye view

- Before your little one begins to crawl, get his point of view of things. Get down on your hands and knees and make a room-by-room crawling tour of your home. Look for things you would never notice from where you stand, such as a long lamp cord, a dangerous stairway, and so on.

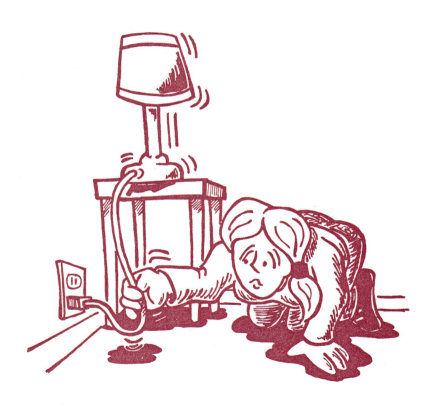

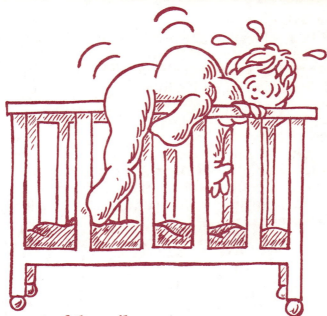

Climbing out of the crib

- When he starts, place a sturdy chair alongside it to help him get down safely. Train him to report to you as soon as he's out of the crib.

- And, be sure to let the crib gate down. This way he can't release it himself and risk being struck as it falls.

Bumper guard

- Make a bumper for baby's walker by slitting pieces of garden hose lengthwise and fitting them over the metal bars. The rubber protects furniture and woodwork from scratches.

Fire safety
- Check all smoke-alarm batteries once a week.

- Buy a fire extinguisher for your house. Check it once a year to make sure it's in good working order.

Tot finder decals
- Stick "tot finder" decals on the outside of nursery windows and along the bottom of the nursery door. In case of fire, the decals help firemen locate your child's room more quickly. (Decals are available at your local fire department.)

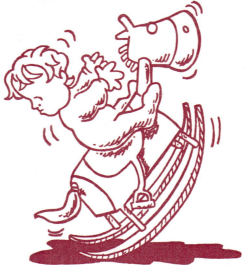

No tipping
- To prevent a child's rocker or rocking horse from tipping, tack a cork to the end of each rocker arm.

Safety steps
- Make sure staircases are well lit.

- Show a toddler how to crawl backwards downstairs. It's safer and easier.

- A carpeted stairway helps prevent a child from slipping, and it cushions the fall if he does.

- When baby is first learning to walk, put safety gates at the top and bottom of the stairs. But remember, he may soon learn to climb over them.

- Teach him that toys are not to be left on the staircase.

Avoiding shocks
- Cover electrical outlets with plastic safety covers (available at hardware stores).

- Move furniture in front of sockets so baby can't get at them.

Power tools
- Wire all workshop power tools into a master switch that's out of the reach of children. When you leave the workshop, flip the switch so that nothing can be turned on.

Window pains
- Windows should have gates, screens or window guards.

Furniture safety
- Before you know it, baby will be climbing on things, so don't place any furniture near a window.

- To protect little fingers, place a cork at each end of a toy box or piano keyboard cover. If the lid drops, there's no need to worry.

- Make sure all valuable and breakable knickknacks are out of your child's reach.

- Covers for sharp table corners can be purchased at hardware stores.

Fan fare
- A safe fan is one that's out of reach.

- To further prevent danger, sew a bag out of some nylon net and fit it over your fan. The bag will also help keep the fan dust-free.

Busy signals
- Use a wide rubber band to hold the contact buttons down. Even if the receiver is pulled off the hook, you can still receive calls.

Comings and goings
- Your toddler will have a hard time sneaking outside if you tie a small bell to the door.

- Or, attach a little bell to your toddler's shoes and you'll be able to keep track of his whereabouts.

Behind closed doors
- Any door can be locked by installing a hook and eye screw out of a child's reach.

- Places like basements, attics, and workshops can be hazardous for curious toddlers. If you don't already have locks on the doors, put a circle of satin, silk, or some other slippery fabric over the doorknob. Make a drawstring to gather the edges around the knob, making it too slippery for little hands to turn.

Glass door hazard
- To prevent a youngster from walking into a glass door, place a piece of colored tape on the glass at child's eye-level.

Preventing lock-ins
- To prevent children from getting locked in a room, drive a small nail in the top of the door trim and hang the key on it.

- Drape a towel over the top of the bathroom door to keep a child from locking himself in.

In the kitchen
- Fold tablecloth edges up on top of the table out of your child's reach.

- Keep dishware and utensils in the middle of the table.

- Sharp knives should be kept out of a toddler's reach, instead of with other utensils in a drawer.

- Cabinets will be impossible to open if you insert a yardstick through the drawer handles.

- If your child likes to play with the oven controls, remove them when not in use.

- Turn pot handles toward the inside of the stove to prevent them from being knocked off.

Bathroom precautions
- Right before bathing, take the phone off the hook. That way, you won't be called away while your child is in the bathroom alone.

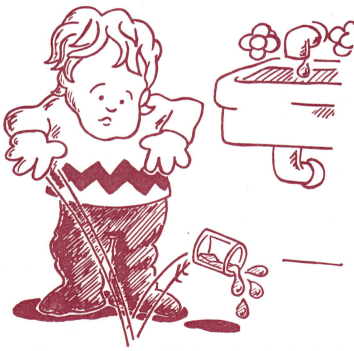

- Paper cups are safer than glass in the bathroom.

- Mark the hot water faucet with red nail polish and teach children the difference.

Appliance cords
- A dangling appliance cord is a dangerous temptation. When not in use, unplug it, roll it up and fasten it with a twist tie or rubber band.

- Or, stuff the cord in an empty toilet tissue tube and tuck it in the back of the appliance.

Poisons
- Write the number of your local poison control center, police, fire department, pediatrician, hospital and pharmacy by every phone in the house.

- Keep whatever shouldn't be swallowed—whether it's liquor, lacquer, medicine or cleaning fluids—out of a child's reach or under lock and key.

Holiday hazards
- Poinsettias, holly berries, and mistletoe may look very appealing to small children but they are poisonous if swallowed. Keep them out of reach.

Shattered glass
- The best solution is your vacuum. But to make sure you get all the pieces, dampen some napkins or paper towels and wipe up the splinters that the broom and dustpan miss.

For proud parents
- Avoid using a direct flash when taking photos of new-born infants. It can cause eye damage.

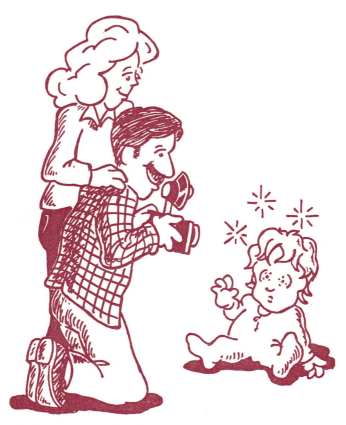

Out of sight, out of mind
- Make sure plastic garbage bags are out of reach of little hands.

- If you have an unused refrigerator or freezer, get rid of it.

- Or, remove the doors.

Walk, don't run
- When a child has a lollipop or popsicle—anything with a stick—enforce a "No running" rule.

Yard guard
- Police your yard for pebbles, glass, sticks and other debris that can fly out of the lawn mower.

- And, when mowing, keep children away.

If your kid's a swinger
- Put a heavy coat of paint on a swing seat to avoid splinters.

- Non-slip bathtub strips affixed to the seat will prevent him from slipping off.

- Cover swing chains with sleeves made from an old garden hose. This will protect clothes from catching in the links, and provide a firmer grip.

One more look around the house
- For safety's sake, remove the push buttons on top of aerosol cans before throwing them away. The cans will be unsprayable should little hands get hold of them.

- Tie a knot in the bottom of plastic cleaning bags hanging in your closet. This will prevent a curious toddler from sticking his head inside the open end.

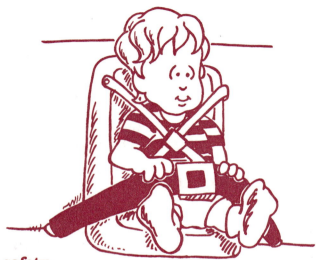

Car safety
- Starting with the very first ride home from the hospital, the infant should be secured in a car safety seat. It's the law in many states!

- Never leave children alone in a car.

Avoiding an identity crisis
- When taking a toddler shopping or to a crowded place, write your name and address on a piece of adhesive tape and stick it on the instep of his shoe. Explain that he should show the tape to someone if he gets lost.

When Baby's Not Well

We've all had the sniffles, colds and the flu,
Chances are baby will have them too
But don't let it throw you for a loop...
It's time to make good chicken soup!

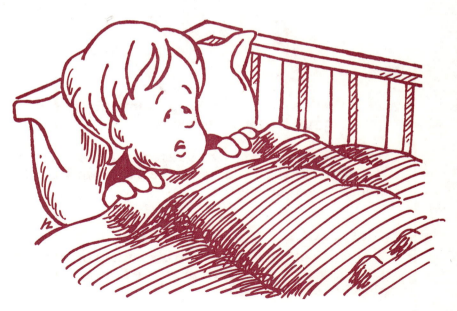

Temperature taking

- Remember, a rectal thermometer registers a fever within 30 to 45 seconds after insertion.

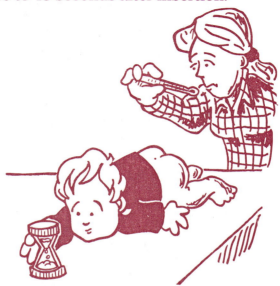

- An egg timer will help you keep your youngster occupied while you take her temperature.

- Don't shake down the thermometer until the next use. If you have to call the doctor, there'll be no mistake in reporting the temperature.

New prescriptions

- When you call the doctor, have previously prescribed medicines in front of you. It may save time and money ordering new prescriptions.

76

Medicines and vitamins

- Store infant medications, vitamins and measuring spoons in a spice rack inside a locked kitchen cupboard. Everything's within easy reach for you, but out of reach of little children.

- Medicine bottles, spoons and other utensils are easier to carry to the sick bed if you put them inside a bread loaf pan.

- Keep track of the times you give medication. This is especially important when two or more are involved. Set an alarm clock to remind you.

- Before reusing old medicines, consult your doctor.

If it's hard to swallow

- Baby will take even the worst-tasting medicine if you put the prescribed amount in a nipple and give it to her right before feeding time.

- Desensitize tastebuds by letting your youngster suck on an ice cube before giving her bad-tasting medicine.

- If she has trouble swallowing a pill, crush it into a teaspoon of applesauce.

Mixing medicine

- It's not a good idea to mix medicine with a bottle of juice or formula. If baby doesn't drink it all, he won't get the full dose and you won't know how much was taken.

Spooning it out

- Avoid spills by giving baby medicine in a medicine dropper.

- When giving a spoonful of medicine to your toddler, have her hold an empty paper cup under her chin. This helps prevent spills and you can keep track of how much medicine actually goes down.

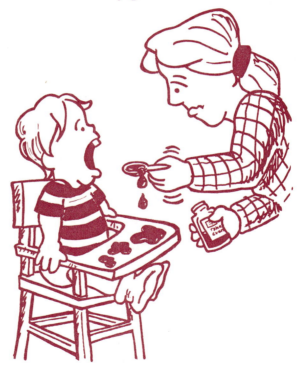

- Or, when the prescription calls for one teaspoon, pour that amount into a tablespoon.

- Bath time is the best time to give your child liquid vitamins. Baby is more relaxed, and if anything spills, there'll be nothing to launder.

Eyedrops and eardrops without teardrops
- While your child is lying down with his eyes closed, place the eyedrops in the corner of each eye. When he opens them, the drops will spread evenly throughout.

- Set a bottle of eardrops in warm water for a few minutes before using.

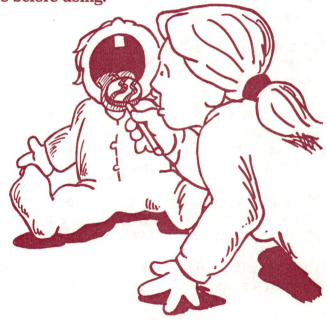

Open up and say, "Ahhh"
- A lollipop makes a delicious tongue depressor.

Cool-mist vaporizer
• Direct the mist where you want it to go by taping a 3-foot length of vent pipe to the vaporizer opening.

Why baby "runs"
• If you sterilize formula, you may be evaporating too much water, making the formula more concentrated than it should be. This can cause diarrhea. Instead, use the bottom rack of the dishwasher for sterilizing bottles and add boiled water to the formula. That might do away with the problem.

Winterizing your toddler
• To prevent frost-nipped cheeks, apply a light coat of petroleum jelly.

Bruises, burns and cuts
• Keep a few red washclothes or napkins handy to clean minor cuts. The sight of blood won't be as noticeable or traumatic for either of you.

• Don't apply antiseptic salve directly to a cut. Put it on the bandage and then apply it to the skin. It doesn't seem to hurt as much that way.

• A band-aid will come off without the hurt if you first rub it with a piece of cotton soaked in baby oil.

• When baby is learning to walk, keep an ice-cube tray filled with frozen juice. If she falls and bumps her lip, the cubes are a tasty way to reduce the swelling.

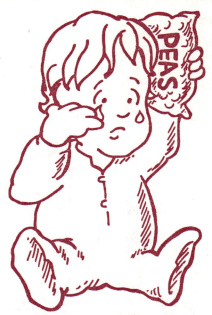

- In a pinch, a plastic bag filled with frozen, uncooked peas makes a flexible compress.

Splinters
- If you can't pinpoint the splinter, dab on a little iodine. The splinter will turn dark and be easy to locate.

- To remove the splinter, soak it in cooking oil for a few minutes. It should loosen and be easy to remove.

- Or, apply an ice cube to the finger for a few minutes to numb the area before removal.

- A little teething lotion may do the same trick.

Teething treats

- Popsicles are soothing to baby's gums.

- Freeze some yogurt in an ice-cube tray; then cut the cubes into bite-size pieces.

- Freeze bananas and let the teether suck on them.

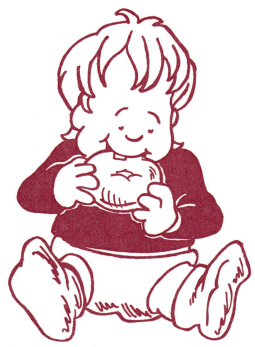

- Or, give him a frozen bagel.

Teething tricks

- A cold, wet towel feels good on baby's gums.

- On those drooling days, have her wear a bib all day to absorb the moisture.

- Make sure nipple holes of bottles are large enough at this time. Strenuous sucking further irritates sore and swollen gums.

- Keep several teething rings in the refrigerator so replacements are ready when she needs them.

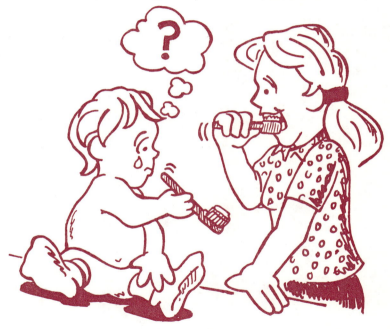

- If you're having trouble applying numbing solution to swollen gums, put some on a toothbrush. Let her apply it while she watches you brush your teeth.

Cleaning baby's teeth

- Help keep plaque away by wiping teeth and gums with a washcloth.

Keeping health records

- For easy access, keep medical information with the birth certificate.

Playing Around

Building blocks, wind-up clocks
Are put aside when baby spots a box...
Parents, it's time to smarten,
Don't buy a toy, give him a carton

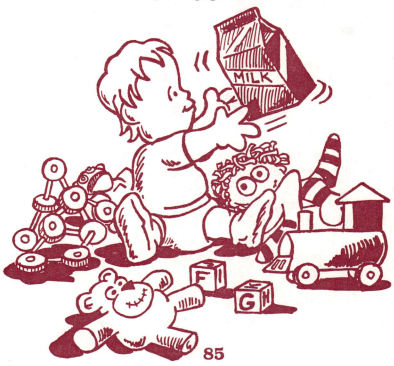

85

Toy safety

- Anything smaller than a baby's fist is not a toy. It could be dangerous! The same goes for big toys with small parts or parts that can be broken off easily.

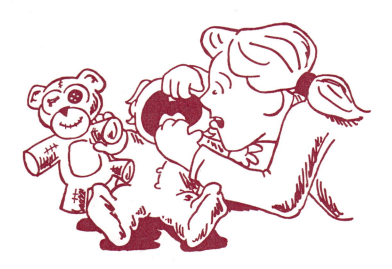

- Steer clear of toys with cords longer than a foot. It doesn't take long to become entangled.

- Opt for embroidered eyes on stuffed toys, not button-type eyes that can be swallowed.

- Squeeze soft toys to make sure there are no wires or pins hidden in the fabric.

- Plastic riding toys with seamed wheels are hazardous. The seams can split, sending the rider for a nasty spill.

- Listen to noise-making toys before you buy them. Shrill sounds can injure a child's hearing — and jangle Mommy's nerves!

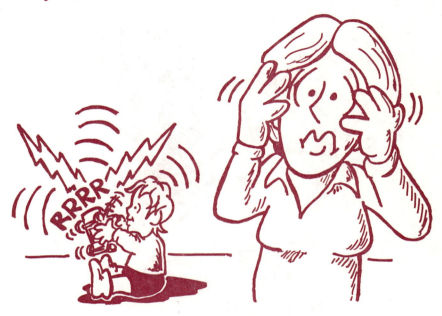

Mobiles
- A plastic hanger makes a good foundation from which to create a mobile.

- Hang an inflatable beach ball over baby's crib. The bright spinning colors will keep baby's attention.

Measure for Measure
- Plastic measuring cups, measuring spoons and bowls are safe, unbreakable toys.

- Make a set of safe blocks by taping the bottom halves of two milk containers and covering them with contact paper.

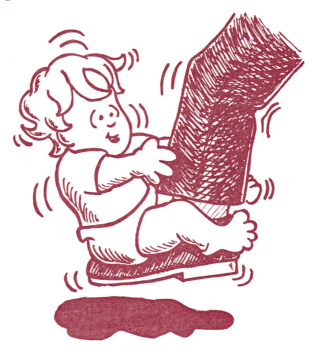

- You will soon find out that baby's favorite toy is you!

In the pen
- Use a plastic inflatable swimming pool as a playpen for a very young child.

- If your child keeps falling down in the playpen, it might be because the mat is slipping. Glue strips of VELCRO Fastener to the corners of the baseboard and attach corresponding strips of fastener to the bottom of the mat. That ought to hold it.

- Use dental floss for mending holes or tears in the playpen netting. It's strong and blends well with the existing mesh.

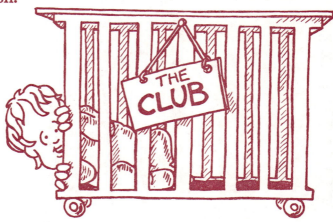

Recycling a playpen
- When your toddler outgrows the playpen, turn it into a clubhouse. Cover the top with a sheet of plywood and remove the slats from one side.

"Weave" me alone
- Knot a shoelace at one end and give it to your child along with a colander. He'll love weaving the lace in and out of the holes. But watch out for any rough edges on the colander!

Modeling clay

- Make your own: Mix 1 cup of salt and 2 cups of flour; add enough water to make the dough soft and pliable and add food coloring. When not in use, it will stay fresh if you keep it tightly sealed in a plastic bag or airtight container.

- To soften hardened modeling clay, wrap it in wet paper towel and place in a microwave oven for a few seconds.

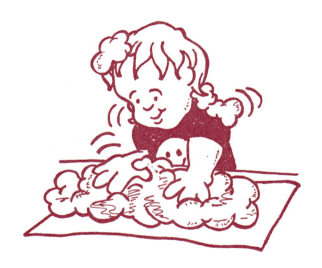

Painting the town

- Make finger paints in your kitchen by mixing 2 cups of cold water and ¼ cup cornstarch. Boil the liquid until thick, then pour into smaller containers and color with food coloring. Allow to cool.

Catching the drips

- Styrofoam egg cartons make ideal containers for finger paints. There's a well for each color and, when the kids are done, just close the lid and throw it away.

- To eliminate messy spills when using a glass as a container, cut an opening in the center of a sponge and insert the glass. The sponge keeps it from tipping over and absorbs any overflow.

- When using store-bought finger paints, add about ¼ teaspoon liquid dishwashing detergents to them. It'll **make spills easier to wipe up.**

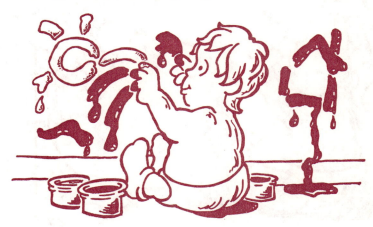

Cleaning the mess

- When your child decides to finger paint the walls and woodwork, first blot up as much paint as possible with a damp rag. Then, gently rub the spot with a damp cloth and baking soda.

- Before trying to wash finger paint off washable fabric, let it dry first. Brush off as much of the paint as you can and launder as you normally would. If any of the stain remains, do not dry the garment in a dryer or the stain will set.

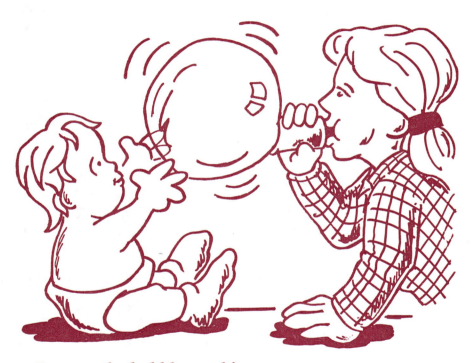

Turn on the bubble machine
- Make your own soap bubbles by mixing liquid soap and water. For big bubbles, cut out the bottom of a small paper cup, dip in a bowl of bubble solution and blow into the top of the cup.

Fresh smooth paste

- To prevent paste from drying out, moisten the lid with water before screwing it back on.

Crayon care

- A dab of all-purpose household cleaner on a moist rag will remove stubborn crayon marks from the new "color and wipe" drawing boards.

- Wrap crayons and chalk with masking tape and there will be less chance of breakage.

- Sharpen your child's crayons by holding the end under hot water to soften the wax, then shape the point with your finger.

Toy storage

- Attach an ice cream bucket to your child's walker as a tag-along toy chest. Tie the handle to a leg with a macrame cord.

- A large plastic laundry basket makes a safe, sturdy toy basket. Turn it upside down and it's a bench for your youngster.

- Or, use a large box of disposable diapers.

More storage ideas

- The bottom of a child's dresser makes a neat, out-of-the-way place to store games and toys. Better yet, when he wants them, he can get them himself.

- Or, use a bookshelf. Make it topple-proof by attaching it to the wall with hook and eye screws or L-braces.

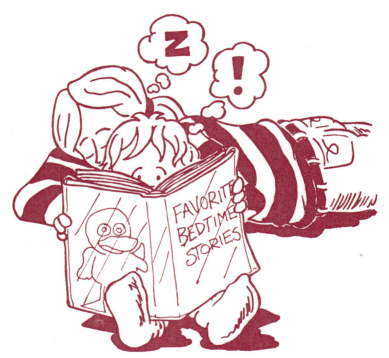

"Cover" stories
- Preserve your youngster's favorite storybooks by covering the pages with clear contact paper.

- And, reinforce the top and bottom covers of game boxes with masking tape to avoid broken corners and lost pieces.

A clean sweep

- After your youngster is through playing with building blocks or toys with lots of pieces, use a broom to sweep all the pieces into one big pile. Then he can pick them up and put them away by himself.

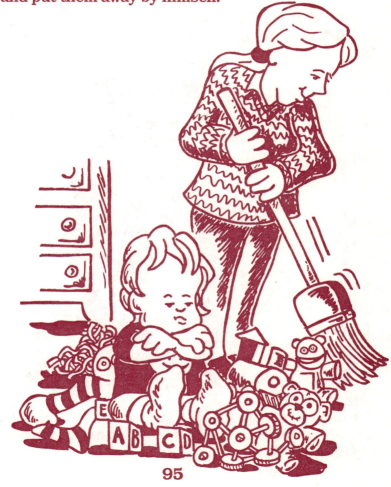

Cleaning two birds with one bath

- Toss rubber and plastic toys in your little one's bath. After the bath is over, rinse with hot water and hang the toys to dry in a nylon net drawstring bag.

- Or, put them in the bag and toss them in the washing machine. Hang to dry.

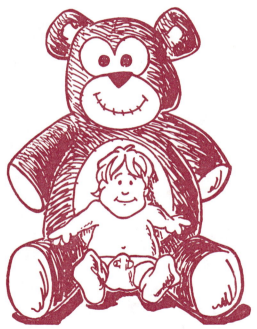

Stuffed toy care

- Try rug shampoo and a stiff brush for cleaning soiled stuffed toys. Dry them on the line and brush to restore original fluffiness.

- Or, clean with dry cornstarch. Rub in, let stand briefly and brush off.

- Stuffed toys with plastic faces should not be put in your dryer. Instead, hang them in sunlight or in a warm area in your home.

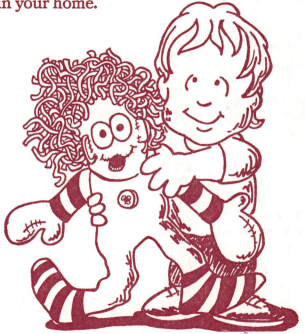

Tangled doll hair
- A bit of fabric softener will help remove tangles from doll's hair. Place a few drops in the palm of your hand, apply to the doll's hair and allow it to set for a moment. Then, dampen the hair with water and you will be able to comb through the knots with ease.

Outdoor toys
- Instead of buying a sandbox, fill a plastic swimming pool with sand.

- To put the "slip" back in a child's slide, rub it down with waxed paper.

Rusty swingset
- To prevent rust, coat the metal parts with car wax several times a year.

Squeaky wheels
- Petroleum jelly is a good lubricant for squeaky tricycle wheels.

Repairing inflatable toys
- To find a pin hole, put the toy in water and look for air bubbles. When you locate it, cover with two or three coats of nail polish. If that doesn't solve the problem, patch the hole with vinyl sealer (available in hardware stores).

And Away We Go

Traveling with baby is a delicate art---
On a long plane ride or in a shopping cart
This chapter is meant to bring out the smiles
As you and your baby cover the miles

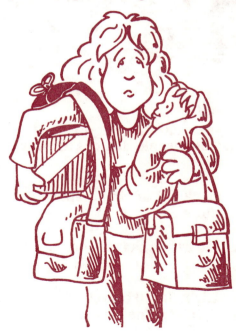

GOING BY CAR

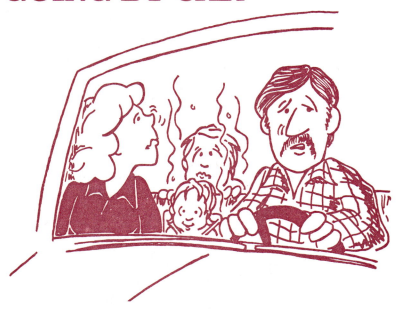

Pack up all your cares and go

- Keep a few disposable diapers in your glove compartment.

- And save space by packing disposable diapers in the corners of suitcases.

- Large plastic garbage bags are handy for stashing soiled laundry.

- Pack a nightlight. It will be a comfort if your child wakes up at night in a strange room.

- And, don't forget to take a foldable, lightweight aluminum stroller. They're a blessing on any trip.

Another space-saving hint
- Take along inflatable toys. Uninflated.

Before taking off
- Don't let your youngster have cola drinks during the trip. The caffeine can make him irritable and jumpy. Caffeine also acts as a diuretic and could add to the number of rest stops you have to make.

- Throw a sheet over the back seat. It will catch crumbs, drips and spills.

Before shutting the door
- After your toddlers have climbed into the car say, "Stick 'em up." With all hands in the air, there's no chance of smashing fingers in the door.

- Make a game out of having the last one in the car be responsible for checking to see that all doors are locked.

- Teach children not to open the door until you hold up the ignition key.

Safety seats
- All children up to the age of four should ride in a child's safety seat. It's best to put it in the back seat.

- Use seat belts to secure baby's safety seat.

- In warm weather, metal parts on safety seats can get very hot. To avoid burned fingers, cover the seat with a fitted cloth cover.

- Or, cover the seat with a terry cloth towel. Remember to cut holes in it for the straps to pass through. The towel will also absorb moisture and help keep baby cool.

- To protect the car's upholstery, put a piece of heavy vinyl carpet runner under the safety seat.

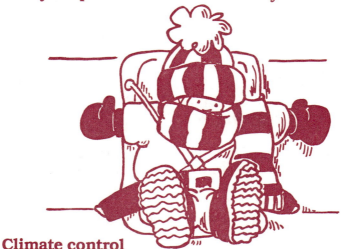

Climate control
- Keep in mind the temperature inside the car. Don't over-dress your child in winter when the heater is on; don't under-dress her in summer when the air conditioner is running.

Bottle storage

- To keep a bottle refrigerated when traveling, put it inside a wide-mouth insulated Thermos bottle with a few chunks of ice. It will stay cool for hours.

- Or, put it inside a locking plastic bag with a few ice cubes. Wrap in a diaper or a dish towel.

Fast food to go

- Instead of traveling with bottles of regular milk, carry powdered milk in the bottles. Just add water and shake.

- Or, pour measured amounts of powdered formula into locking plastic bags and fill a Thermos bottle with warm water. When baby is hungry mix the formula in the warm water.

Bottle warmers

- If you don't plan to stop very often, consider buying a bottle warmer that plugs into the car's cigarette lighter.

- Or, fill a moist towelette container with very hot water and insert the bottle. In three to six minutes, the bottle is the right temperature for baby to drink.

- For shorter trips, heat the bottle before leaving and keep it warm by wrapping in a towel and putting it inside an empty potato chip can. Make sure the can is tightly sealed.

Preventing leaks

- Cover the bottle mouth with a piece of plastic wrap before putting on the nipple and cap. Remove the wrap before feeding.

Travel bib
- A disposable diaper makes an emergency travel bib. Open the diaper and secure with tabs around the baby's neck (soft side in).

Quick cleanup
- Place a wet washcloth or moist towelette in a plastic bag and carry it in your purse or glove compartment.

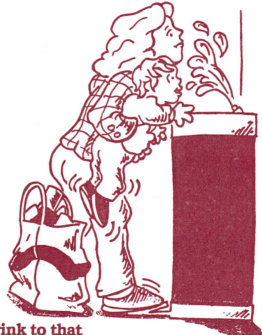

Let's drink to that
- Keep a collapsible cup in your purse. It's much easier to drink from than a water fountain.

- Carry small cans of juice in your car or purse. It's not always convenient to stop when your toddler gets thirsty.

Auto amusements
- Tie elastic or string to small toys, then tie them to the infant car seat. If baby drops her toy, she can retrieve it herself instead of you taking your eyes off the road to do it. Make sure the string or elastic is very secure!

- Soft toys are safest in a car.

- If you have a cassette player or tape deck, buy or make tapes especially for the baby.

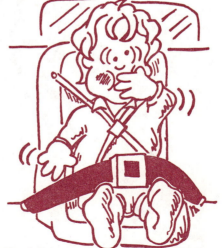

Car sickness
- A high-carbohydrate, low-fat diet a few days before a car trip seems to make it easier on a child who has a tendency to get car sick.

- Set your child high enough in the infant seat so he can look out the front window. Watching scenery pass sideways causes nausea.

- Don't smoke.

- Carry a plastic ice cream container with a lid in case the above precautions fail.

OUT AND ABOUT

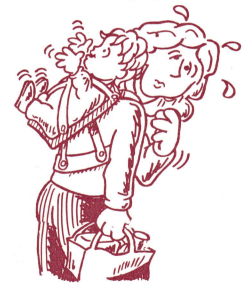

Baby backpacking
- Babies seem happy traveling in back carriers. You can start using them after about five months when your baby's neck is strong enough to take all the jostling.

- Before using a carrier, give yourself plenty of time to build up strength for handling and wearing it.

- If you use the kind of carrier that stands by itself, you can also feed him in it.

- When shopping in a department store, put baby in a carrier. Strollers and crowds don't mix well.

Shopping cart smarts
- Pad the supermarket cart seat with blankets.

- Take your infant seat into the market. Most seats fit into the shopping cart seat.

- Buckle up for safety. Use an adult-size belt around the baby, securing him in the cart.

- Or, use a cloth diaper or a dish towel as a safety belt.

At a restaurant
- If a highchair isn't available, a car seat can usually be used in restaurants.

- Ask your waitress to bring toddler's dinner a few minutes before yours. That gives you a head start on meat cutting, mashing vegetables and other dinnertime chores. Then, when your dinner comes, you can eat in peace.

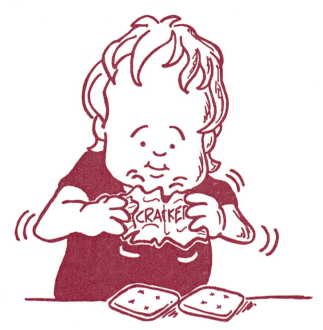

- If your child gets cranky during dinner, ask for a few packages of crackers. The cellophane wrapping may keep him busy long enough for you to eat.

- You'll never be caught without a bib if you keep a sweater chain in your purse. Use it to clip a napkin around your youngster's neck, like the dentist does.

At the movies
- Bring booster seats when you take the kids to the movie or other sit-down events. They'll be able to see all the action.

Changing in the car

- Do you find it a hassle to change diapers on your car's slanted seat? Keep a covered box in the trunk with everything necessary for changing, including a folded blanket. Park the car and change the baby from the trunk where there's plenty of room and everything's right at hand.

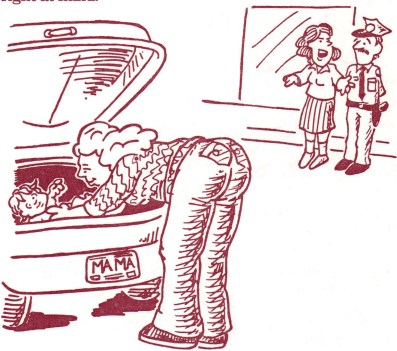

At the beach

- A sunburn is dangerous and avoidable. Turn a playpen upside down, put up an umbrella, or stay for only a short time if there's not enough shade.

109

- Take a plastic laundry basket to the beach. It's a good way to carry things from the car to the sand and back.

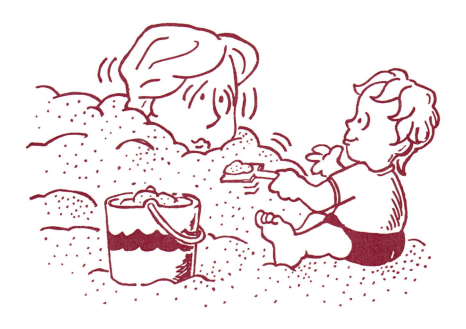

- A big sheet will be cooler than a blanket for you and baby to sit on. It shakes clean easier, too.

- Beach toys in a mesh bag can be dunked in the water to clean and drain dry.

- If you're taking the playpen to the beach, bring along four large jar lids to place under the legs. It keeps them from sinking into the sand.

Away on a visit

- If you visit someone frequently, like Grandma, leave an extra bottle, nipple, box of diapers and a few toys. No sense carting these necessities back and forth.

- Bring a large plastic garbage bag with you. Now you don't have to worry when changing the baby on your hostess' antique bedspread.

On the spot

- Carry some baking soda and a few cotton balls in a plastic bag. If baby spits up, wet a ball, dip it in the baking soda and wipe the soiled area. It's a foolproof cure for "sour smell."

FAR AWAY

In a motel

- Need a bed for baby? Use a blanket-lined drawer.

- If you don't want to rent a crib, simply use a small inflatable plastic pool. Blow it up and cover it with a sheet. Secure the ends underneath the pool.

- Or, get a clean, heavy-duty cardboard box. Set it up on the floor and line the bottom with a heavy quilt. The sides will keep drafts off baby.

- Car beds are handy at motels, hotels, and the homes of friends or relatives where sleeping space is at a premium.

Camping out

- The best single piece of baby equipment for camping is a car safety seat with adjustable, reclining positions for sitting, drinking, and napping.

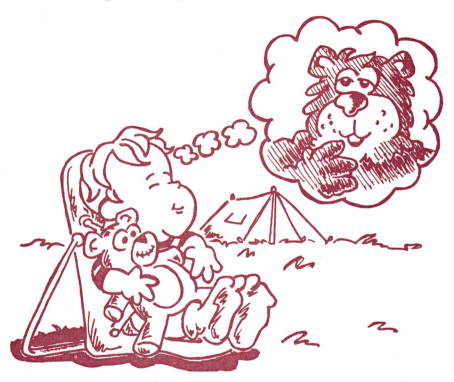

- Create a portable bathtub by inflating a small wading pool.

- For safety sake, dress children in bright-colored clothing.

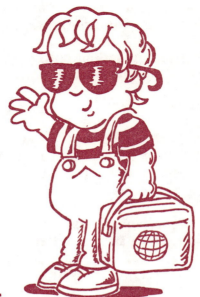

The plane facts
- Children under two years travel free, but are expected to share your seat.

- If you fly during off times, you may be able to set baby on an empty seat next to you, free of charge.

- Airlines do not allow infant seats on board the plane. But you can take a foldable stroller. The hostess will keep it in a cabin closet for you.

Flying high
- During take-offs and landings, give baby a bottle or pacifier to reduce pressure on ears.

- If she takes medication or vitamins, put them in your purse just in case your luggage gets lost.

- Take the air-sickness bag with you. It may come in handy for any number of things while traveling.

Baby abroad
- If you are traveling in Europe, know your baby's weight in kilos (1 kilo = 2.2 pounds; 10 kilos = 22 pounds). Now you'll be able to get the right size disposable diapers in a store.

- Have your doctor prescribe medicines and vitamins you should take for baby in case of minor upsets. The laws in European countries are different from here and, at times, it's even hard to get an aspirin.

Standing In for Mommy and Daddy

Before you leave the sitter with baby
You cover every "if", "but", or "maybe."
Repeat the instructions, one after another,
Isn't it fun when your sitter's your mother?

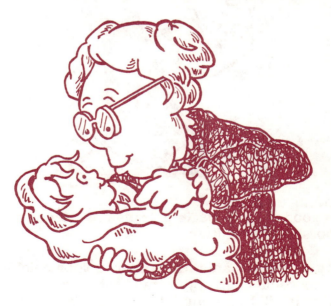

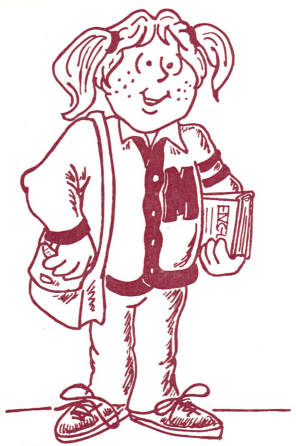

Finding a sitter
- A good place to begin is by asking friends and neighbors to refer a sitter.

- There may be another mother in your neighborhood who would be happy to trade baby-sitting duties with you. It will be helpful if the babies are close in age.

- Baby sitters looking for work sometimes advertise on local bulletin boards. Also, check for listings at high schools, college placement offices and churches.

- Or, get in touch with your local YW/YMCA or 4-H Club. These organizations sometimes offer sitter training programs for teenagers, making it possible for you to find a qualified young person.

Sitter swapping
- Contact other parents in your neighborhood and form a baby-sitter co-operative. Pool the names of sitters, including the hours they are available to work and their rates. This way, you'll have a choice of sitters to call when you need one.

Interviewing the sitter
- When you are trying to find the most qualified person to care for your child, don't be shy about asking for references. Follow up by calling on those references to get their impressions of the sitter.

- Discuss and settle on a fair rate of pay.

Telephone instructions
- It's important that your sitter know how to answer the telephone properly. For example, a sitter should say that you can't come to the phone rather than telling callers that you are out of the house.

- Have a pad and pencil handy for taking phone messages.

117

The best test

- During the interview, excuse yourself for a few minutes and give the sitter time alone with your child. Station yourself in an inconspicuous place so you can hear how baby and the sitter react to each other. It may provide the best clues as to how they would get along when you're not home.

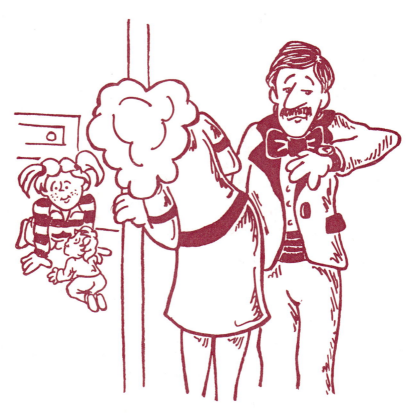

Every sitter should know

- Before leaving, be sure to write down the following information:
  - ☐ The place you are going, including the address and telephone number
  - ☐ The time you expect to be home
  - ☐ Neighbor's name and number
  - ☐ Doctor's name and number
  - ☐ Police and fire emergency number
  - ☐ Poison control center number

Diaper changing

- If you're a little nervous about having the sitter change baby's diapers on the vanity or changing table, arrange to have the sitter do it on the floor. Have a lap pad ready to place under the baby.

Getting acquainted

- Here's a nice way to break the ice: Give the sitter something to give to your child. A new toy or favorite snack usually work well.

- And, to make the sitter feel at home, prepare a light snack or show her around the kitchen and tell her she can make her own.

For baby's sake

- If you put your youngster to bed before the sitter arrives, tell her the sitter is coming so she won't be frightened if she wakes to find you're not there.

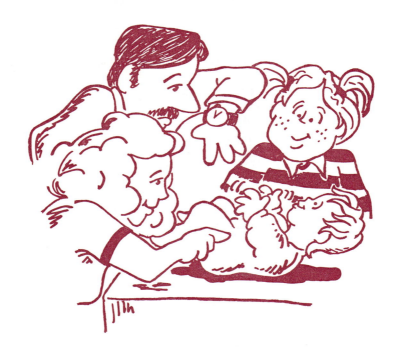

- And, be sure to say good-night before you leave, reassuring her that you'll be back soon.

Miscellaneous Mommying Hints

These are hints
Your mother isn't tellin'
Unless, of course,
Your mom is Mary Ellen

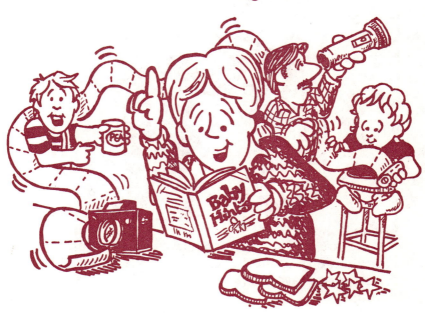

SIBLING JEALOUSY

Preparing an older child

- If big brother or sister is going to be moved to another room because of the new baby, make the change several weeks before the due date. Make it seem like a "promotion" for the "big boy or girl".

- If possible, start your older child at nursery school long before baby's arrival. Don't have her think of school as a way to get rid of her because of the new baby.

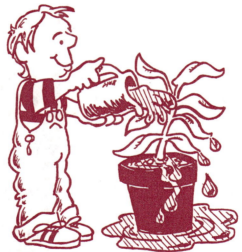

At the hospital

- Make your at-home child feel important by placing him in charge of something while you're away. Have him water your favorite plant or take care of a personal belonging.

- Make special calls to your child without talking to any-one else.

- Remember to refer to the newborn as "our baby".

Greetings from baby

- Prepare a gift for the older child before you leave for the hospital. After the birth, mail it to him along with a snapshot and "greetings" from the new baby brother or sister.

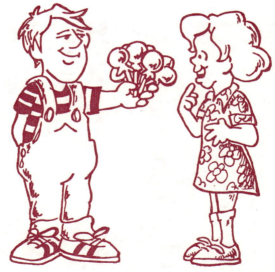

Birthday celebration

- Buy a box of bubble gum cigars and lollipops and tie colorful ribbons around them. When the baby is born, have your older child pass them out to friends, just like Daddy hands out cigars.

Preventing jealousy at home

- On occasion, make time to spend with your older child. Take her to lunch or to a movie, or work on a project together—something having nothing to do with baby.

- When visitors come, let her share in showing them the new family addition.

- If big sister competes for attention while you're talking to baby, make her the topic of conversation and both children will be happy.

TRICKS OF THE TRADE

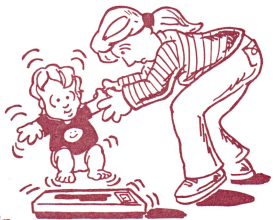

Weighing in

- Here's how to watch your weight while keeping track of baby's: Weigh yourself on the bathroom scale, then weigh yourself while holding baby in your arms. Baby's weight is the difference between the two.

Pacifiers in a pinch

- If you can't find any of baby's pacifiers, use a bottle nipple instead. That should hold him till one turns up.

- To prevent a pacifier from falling on the floor or getting lost in the car, tie a ribbon to it and fasten through a zipper pull or button loop.

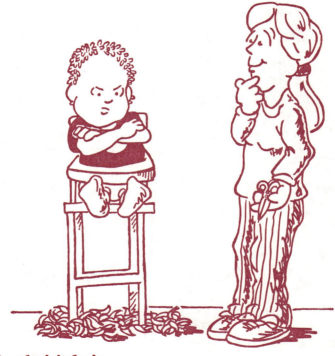

Cutting heir's hair

- Hair won't fall in his face if you tape a piece of wax paper under his bangs.

Toying with your toddler

- Stash a few of your tot's toys in a dresser drawer. Bring them out when you want to keep him busy while you finish dressing.

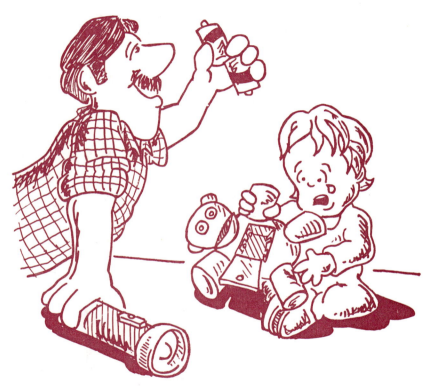

Batteries not included

- Always keep an emergency candle on hand. If the lights go out, you can find the toys that have the batteries which were borrowed from the flashlight!

Tricks at the table

- When you're almost out of bread and your youngster won't eat a sandwich made with the crust, flip it over so the white part is on the outside. She'll never know the difference.

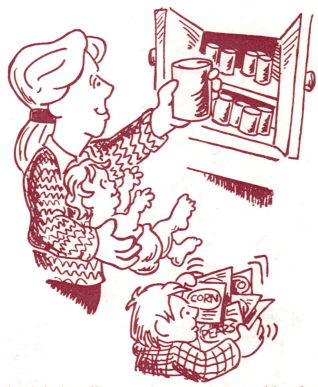

- Take the labels off several canned vegetables before storing them in the cupboard. When the kids argue about which vegie to have at dinner, settle it by opening one of the mysterious, unmarked cans.

Potty training

- Training little boys to use the toilet is a lot easier if they sit on the seat backwards, facing the tank. They can hang onto the tank without fear of falling in, and everything goes where it's supposed to go.

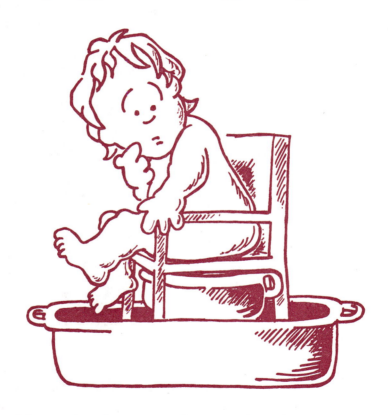

- A large aluminum roasting pan placed under the potty chair will catch any "misses".

A star is born

- Frustrated by your toddler's potty training progress? Maybe he needs a reward for a job well done. Tape a piece of paper on the wall next to the potty chair and put a box of brightly-colored stars on a shelf nearby. After each successful attempt, let your child pick out a star and stick it on the paper. He'll be proud of his accomplishments and soon, he'll be a "star" in the bathroom by himself.

Spin-offs

- Little children seem to enjoy spinning toilet tissue off the roll. To eliminate spin-offs, squeeze the roll together so it's no longer round before inserting it on the spindle.

Throwing in the towel

- Put some VELCRO Fastener on the edges of a few old towels. Loop the towels around the towel rack and fasten, allowing most of the towel to hang down. Your toddler can wipe his hands and face without pulling the towel onto the floor.

Photo genius

- When taking your child to a professional photographer, bring along a favorite stuffed toy. With all the commotion and bright lights, the toy will be a comfort and he won't be as nervous.

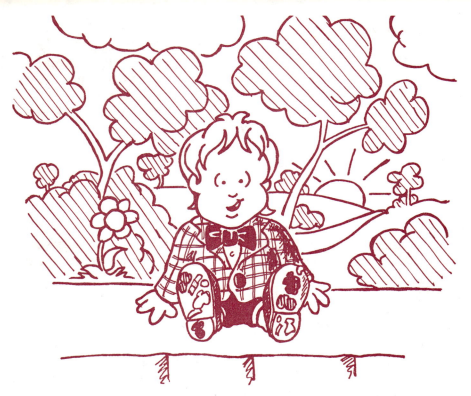

- Be sure to wash the bottom of your toddler's shoes before professional photos are taken. Kids are almost always posed sitting with their legs folded and the bottom of the shoes will show.

- Once a year, every year, take a picture of your child in the same location and pose: in front of a tree in the yard; at the front door; sitting at the piano. It will be a treasured history of growth in pictures.